50th Birthday Guest Book
50 blank pages

rag id
SEO

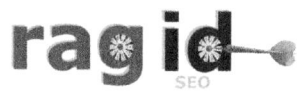

ISBN-13: 978-1539026549
ISBN-10: 153902654X
Copyright 2016 by RAGID-Selbstverlag
Kontaktdaten siehe www.ragid.de
1. Auflage

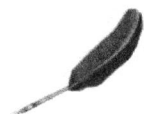

50th Birthday

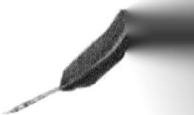

50th Birthday

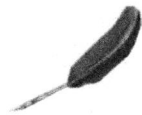

50th Birthday

50th Birthday

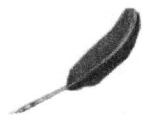

50th Birthday

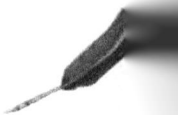

50th Birthday

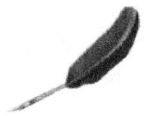

50th Birthday

50th Birthday

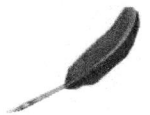

50th Birthday

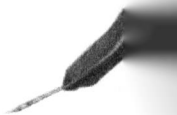

50th Birthday

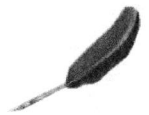

50th Birthday

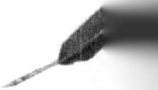

50th Birthday

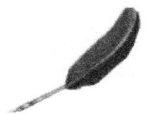

50th Birthday

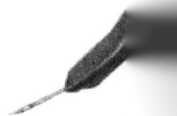

50th Birthday

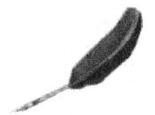

50th Birthday

50th Birthday

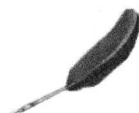

50th Birthday

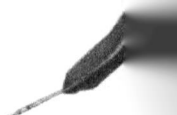

50th Birthday

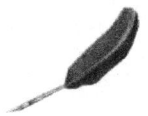

50th Birthday

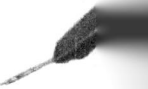

50th Birthday

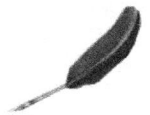

50th Birthday

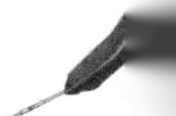

50th Birthday

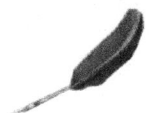

50th Birthday

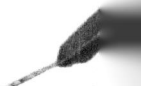

50th Birthday

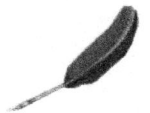

50th Birthday

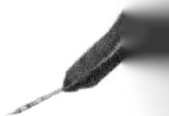

50th Birthday

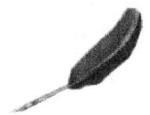

50th Birthday

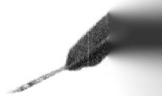

50th Birthday

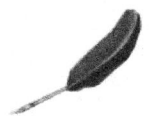

50th Birthday

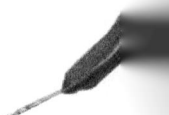

50th Birthday

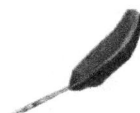

50th Birthday

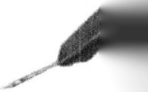

50th Birthday

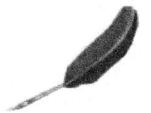

50th Birthday

50th Birthday

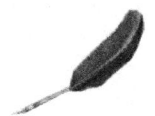

50th Birthday

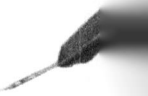

50th Birthday

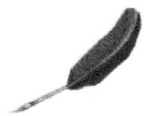

50th Birthday

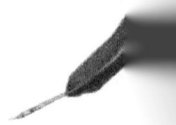

50th Birthday

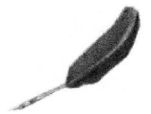

50th Birthday

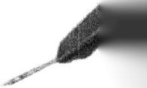

50th Birthday

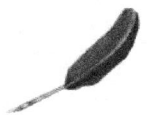

50th Birthday

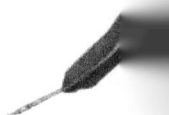

50th Birthday

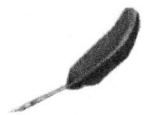

50th Birthday

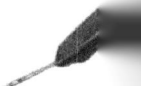

50th Birthday

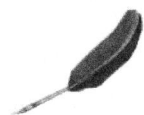

50th Birthday

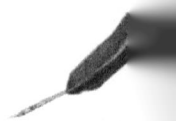

50th Birthday

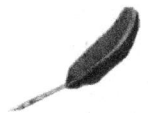

50th Birthday

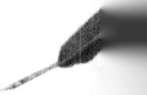

50th Birthday

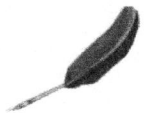

50th Birthday

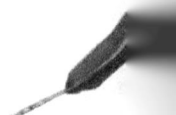

50th Birthday